THE TEETH, JAW AND PERIODONTAL

A COMPENDIOUS STUDY OF THE TEETH, JAW AND PERIODONTAL DEVELOPMENT

Dr. Lynda Charles

THE TEETH, JAW AND PERIODONTAL DEVELOPMENT

ISBN: 9798846298194

DEDICATION

This book is dedicated to God Almighty for his infinite Grace and my lovely mum who has given me every support needed.

TABLE OF CONTENTS

INTRODUCTION

Teeth and jaws constitute a model of the evolutionary developmental biology concept of modularity and they have been considered the key innovations underpinning a classic example of adaptive radiation. However, their evolutionary origins are much debated. Placoderms comprise an extinct clade or grade, to the clade containing chondrichthyans and osteichthyans, and although they clearly possess jaws. Previous studies have suggested that they lack teeth, that they possess convergent evolved tooth-like structures, or that they possess true teeth. Here we use synchrotron radiation X-ray tomographic microscopy (SRXTM) of a developmental series of Compagopiscis croucheri (Arthrodira) to show that placoderm jaws are composed of distinct cartilages and gnathal ossifications in both jaws, and a dermal element in the lower jaw. The gnathal ossification is a composite of distinct teeth that developed in succession, polarized along three distinct vectors, comparable to tooth families. The teeth are composed of dentine and bone, and show a distinct pulp cavity that is infilled centripetally as development proceeds.

Jawbones and teeth originate from the first pharyngeal arch and develop in closely related ways. Reciprocal epithelial-mesenchymal interactions are required for the early patterning and morphogenesis of both tissues. Here we review the cellular contribution during the development of the jaw bones and teeth. The maxilla and mandible together form the lower part of the facial skeleton, which performs important functions in our daily life.

The jaw bones serve as anchors for the teeth, which are critical for mastication and speech. In vertebrates, the maxilla and mandible, like most of the other craniofacial bones, are derived from cranial neural crest cells (CNCCs). These cells are known for their multipotency and their extensive migration through the embryo.

CHAPTER ONE

DEVELOPMENT OF THE TEETH.

Tooth development and growth also known as odontogenesis is the complex process of formation of the tooth from embryonic cells, which erupt and integrate into the surrounding tissues in the mouth.

As living things are forming, they go through a developmental process to reach maturity or the final outcome. When teeth are in the *odontogenesis* phase (tooth formation) they go through three developmental periods called categories: growth, calcification, and eruption. The term emergence describes the tooth as it breaks through the gingival tissue.

The development of the tooth entails:

1. Initiation
2. Proliferation
3. Histo-differentiation
4. Morpho-differentiation
5. Apposition

The 1st structure to appear is the enamel organ(6th-8th week utero).

STAGES OF TOOTH DEVELOPMENT

Dental development usually begins in the fifth or sixth week of prenatal life. By the seventh week, epithelial skin cells of the mouth thicken along the ridge of the developing jaws creating a horse-shoe-shaped band called the dental lamina which follows the curve of each developing tooth socket.

The growth period of development is divided into;

1. Epithelial thickening
2. Lamina stage
3. Bud stage
4. Cap stage
5. Bell stage

STAGES OF TOOTH DEVELOPMENT

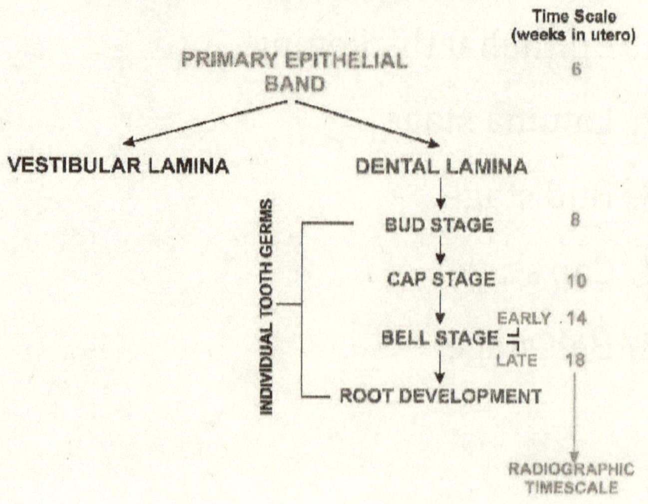

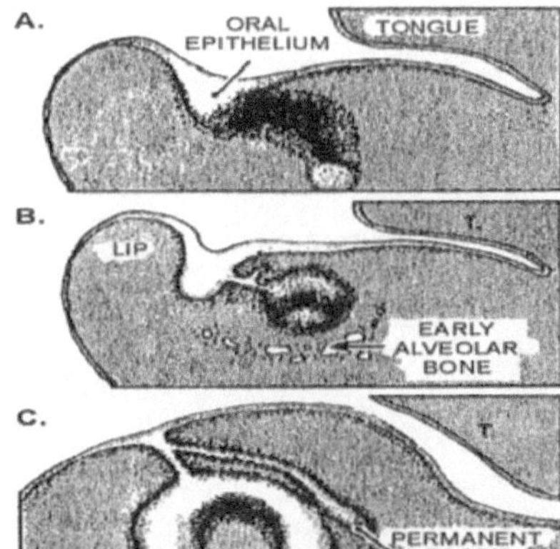

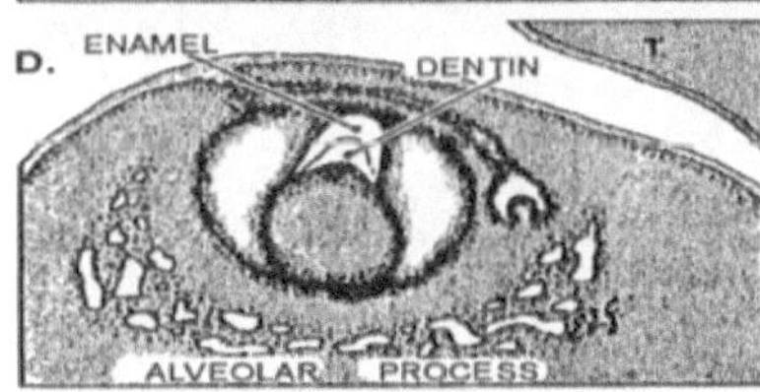

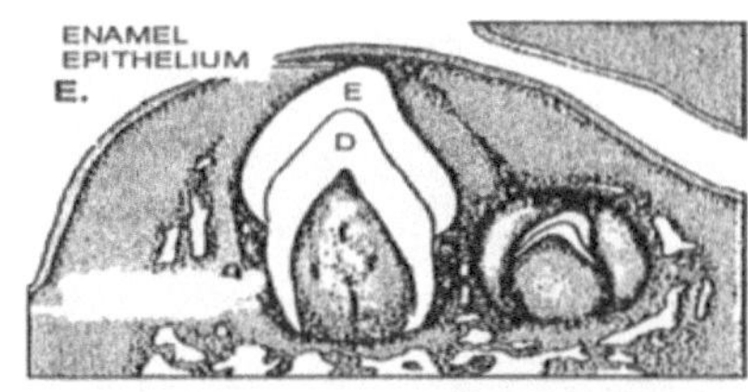

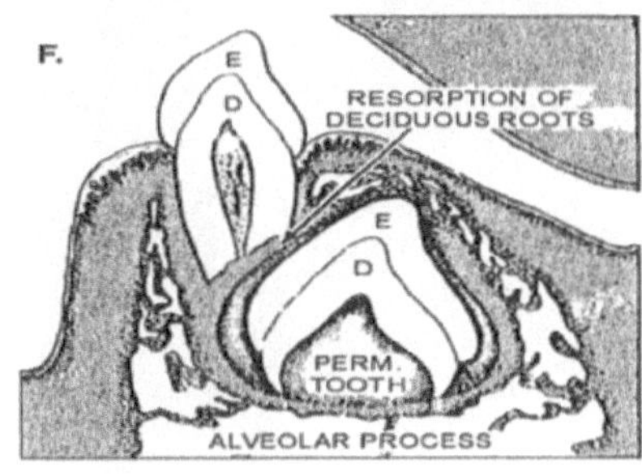

A. BUD STAGE.
B. CAP STAGE.
C. BELL STAGE.
D. CALCIFICATION OF ENAMEL MATRIX.
E. FORMATION OF THE ROOT.
F. RESORPTION OF ROOTS AT DECIDUOUS TOOTH.

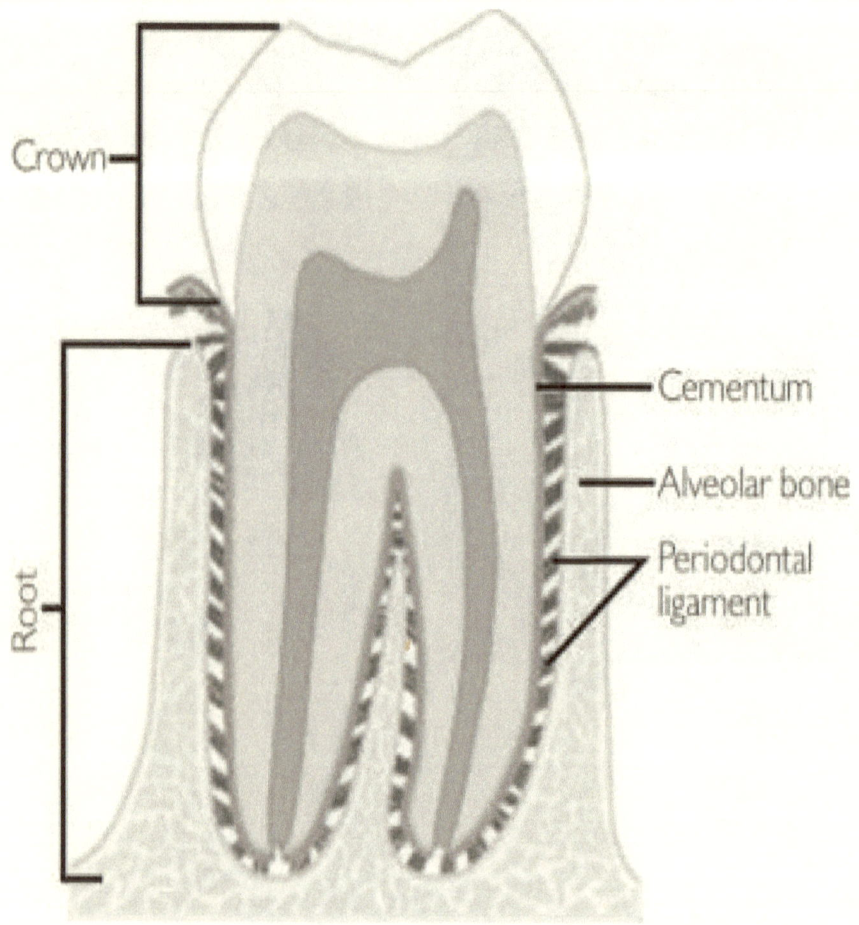
Crown
Root
Cementum
Alveolar bone
Periodontal
ligament

BUD STAGE

As soon as the dental lamina is formed, patches of epithelial cells located there grow into the underlying tissues to become tooth buds. Usually, 10 tooth buds are present in each dental arch and they give rise to future primary teeth. Tooth buds for the permanent teeth form between the 17th week of fetal life through the age of 5 years. When the primary teeth are lost, permanent teeth will replace them.

The proliferation of epithelial ridge from the basal layer of primitive oral epithelium leads to the formation of the dental lamina

20 tooth buds develop as epithelial swellings called enamel organs

Tooth buds are oval or round in shape.

Permanent successors of the deciduous teeth later develop from enamel organs of the inner aspect of deciduous predecessors

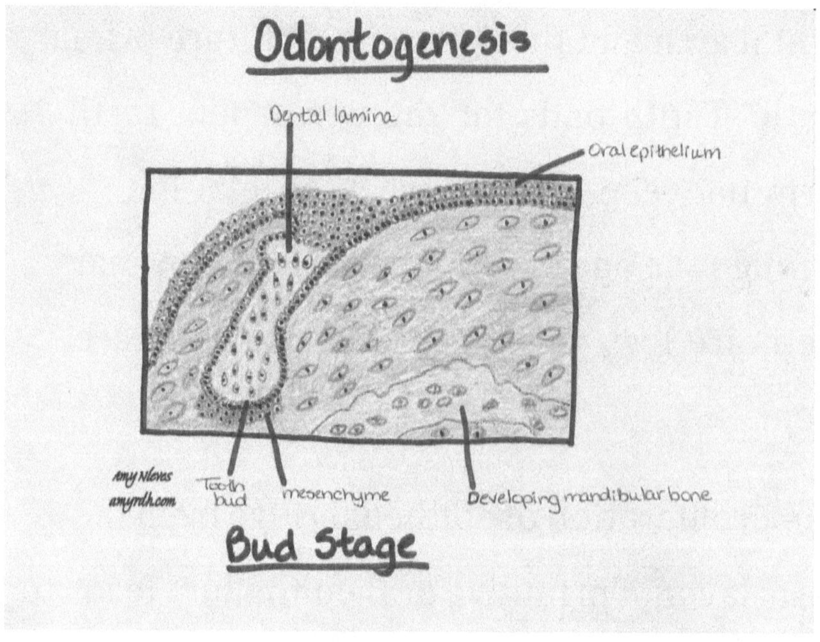

CAP STAGE

This stage is also known as proliferation (reproduction or multiplication) in which the cells of the tooth grow and the tooth bud takes a hollowed cap-like shape. The epithelium of the cap will give rise to the enamel. The zone under the cap is called the dental papilla, a small nipple-shaped elevation. It gives rise to the dentin, cementum, and the pulp.

The basal portion invaginates to enclose the mesenchymal tissue of the dental papilla.

Epithelial cells of the enamel organ differentiate into :

1. External enamel epithelium
2. Internal enamel epithelium

Later, the innermost cells assume star-like shapes and are so-called stellate reticulum.

CAP STAGE

Primordium of the succedaneous tooth
Successful dental lamina
Dental papilla

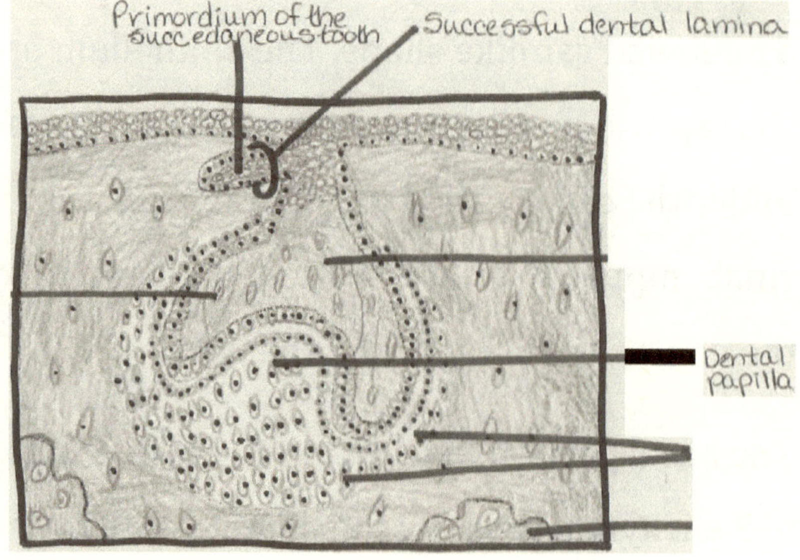

BELL STAGE

The last period of growth is also known as histodifferentiation (the acquisition of tissue characteristics by cell groups) or the bell stage. It is here the ameloblast cells form the enamel, odontoblast cells form the dentin, and the cementoblast cells form the cementum. Concavity in the cap deepens further. Cell layer differentiation – stratum intermedium consisting of flattened cells, 2-3 cells thickens. Dental lamina degenerates into a series of epithelial clumps which may persist – epithelial pearls of Series.

BELL STAGE

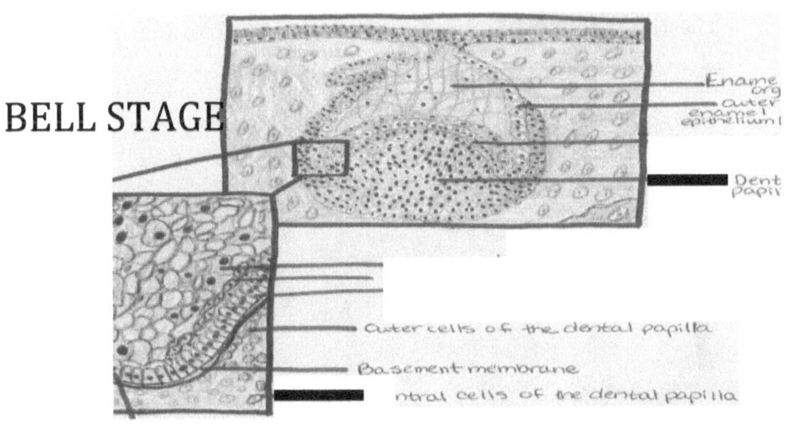

CHAPTER TWO

STRUCTURES OF THE TEETH

A tooth is divided into two parts: the crown and one or more roots

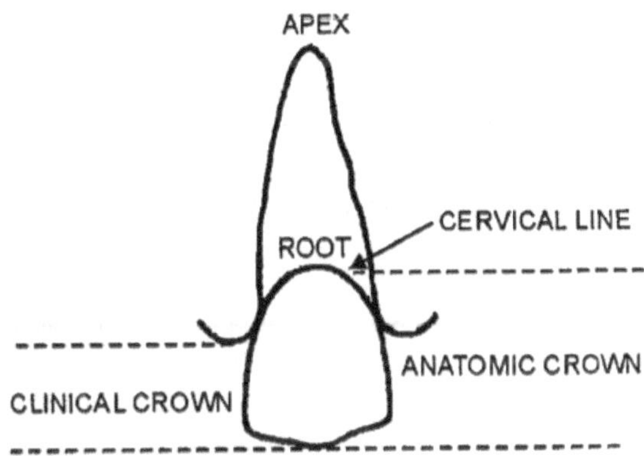

THE CROWN AND THE ROOT

THE CROWN

The crown is divided into the anatomic and clinical crown. The anatomical crown is the portion of the tooth encased in enamel. In young people, areas of the anatomical crown are frequently buried in gingival tissue. As a person gets older, it becomes common for a tooth's enamel to be completely exposed above the gingiva with the root surface showing (gingival recession). The term clinical crown is applied to the part of the crown exposed (visible) in the mouth.

THE ROOT

The root of a tooth is covered by cementum and embedded in a thin layer of compact bone that forms the tooth socket; this is called alveolar bone. The tooth may have a single root or it may have two or three roots. When teeth have more than one root, the region where the roots separate is called the *furcation*. When a tooth has two roots it is bifurcated; when it has three roots it is trifurcated. If a tooth has four or more roots, it is said to be multi-rooted. The tip of each root is called the apex. On the apex of each root, there is a small opening that allows for the passage of blood vessels and nerves into the tooth. This opening is called the apical foramen.

Root Begins to develop after the end of the bell stage of tooth development. The stellate reticulum and the stratum intermedium both degenerate causing the OEE & IEE to lie side by side forming the reduced enamel epithelium. Both OEE & IEE grow apically as two layered epithelial structures called **Hertwig Root Sheath.**

Hertwig's root sheath induces the dental papilla cells adjacent to it to differentiate into odontoblasts – dentine of the root. Hertwig's root sheath begins to break up into fragments called **Epithelial Rest Cells of Malassez.**

Hertwig's root sheath is a proliferation of epithelial cells located at the cervical loop of the enamel organ in a developing tooth. It initiates the formation of dentin in the root of a tooth by causing the differentiation of odontoblasts from the dental papilla. The root sheath eventually disintegrates, but residual pieces that do not completely disappear are seen as **epithelial cell rests of Malassez (ERM).**

Hertwig's sheath is derived from the internal and external enamel epithelium of the enamel organ. The sheath is also responsible for multiple roots (medial growth) and lateral canals (break in epithelium).

Mesenchymal cells from the follicle differentiate into cementoblasts – cementum. The dental follicle gives rise to :

1. Cementum
2. Alveolar bone
3. Collagen fibres of the periodontal membrane

Root formation is completed when dentine formation reduces the funnel-shaped opening of the root apex to a constricted foramen. The time between eruption & root completion for deciduous teeth is about one and half years while for the permanent teeth is about three years.

THE CERVIX

The cervix or cervical line is a slight indentation that encircles the tooth and marks the junction of the anatomical crown with the root. The c e m e n t u m joins the enamel at the cervix of the tooth. The point at which they join is called the cementoenamel junction (CEJ) or cervical line.

TISSUES OF THE TEETH

1. Enamel

2. Dentine

3. Cementum

4. Pulp.

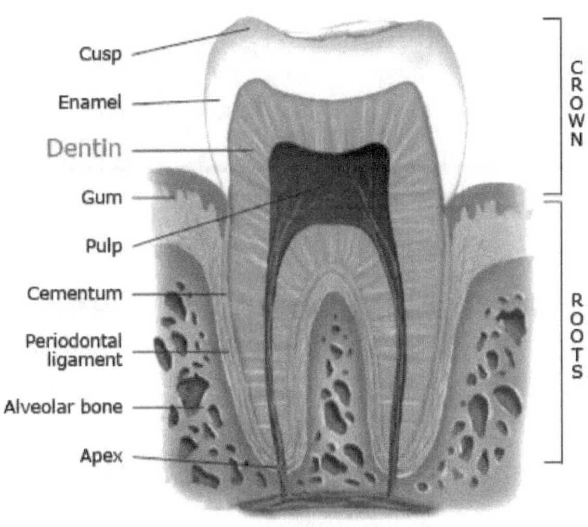

ENAMEL

Enamel is translucent and can vary in color from yellowish to grayish white. The different colors of enamel are attributed to the variation in the thickness, translucent proprieties, the quality of the crystal structure, and surface stains of enamel. Enamel is the calcified substance that covers the entire anatomic crown of the tooth and protects the dentin. Functions as a form of resistant covering of teeth render them suitable for mastication.

It is the hardest tissue in the human body and consists of approximately 96% inorganic minerals, 1% organic materials, and 3% water. Calcium and phosphorus (as hydroxyapatite) are their main inorganic components.

Amelogenesis is the formation of enamel, enamel is formed by epithelial cells (ameloblasts) that lose their functional ability when the crown of the tooth has been completed. After formation, enamel has no power of further growth or repair.

Signals are sent from the newly differentiated odontoblasts to the inner enamel epithelium (IEE), causing the epithelial cells to further differentiate into active secretory ameloblasts.

Amelogenesis has two stages.

1. The first stage is the secretory stage (Proteins and organic matrix form partially mineralized enamel).
2. The second stage is the maturation stage (completes enamel mineralization).

STRUCTURES OF THE ENAMEL

1. Enamel rods
2. Striations

3. Hunter-Schreger bands

4. Incremental lines of Retzius

5. Perikymata

6. Lamellae

7. Neonatal line

8. Enamel cuticle

9. Enamel pellicle

10. Enamel tufts

11. Dentinoenamel junction

12. Odontoblast processes and enamel

FUNCTIONS OF ENAMEL

1. Determines the shape of the crown
2. Initiates dentine formation
3. Establishes the dentinogingival junction
4. Forms enamel

DENTIN

The dentin is a living tissue consisting of specialized cells called odontoblasts and an intercellular substance. Dentin constitutes the bulk of the tooth. Dentin is a light yellow substance that is less dense (radiolucent) than enamel and is very porous; it constitutes the largest portion of the tooth. The pulp chamber is located on the internal surface of the dentin walls. Dentin is harder than bone but softer than enamel. Dentin consists of approximately 70% inorganic matter and 30% organic matter and water. Calcium and phosphorus are their chief inorganic components. Dentin is a living tissue and must be protected during operative or prosthetic procedures from dehydration (drying) and thermal shock.

The dentin is perforated by tubules (similar to tiny straws) that run between the cementoenamel junction (CEJ) and the pulp. Cell processes from the pulp reach part way into the tubules like fingers. These cell processes create new dentin and mineralize it. Dentin transmits pain stimuli by the way of dentinal fibers. Because dentin is a living tissue, it has the ability for constant growth and repair that reacts to physiologic (functional) and pathologic (disease) stimuli.

FORMS OF DENTIN

1. Primary dentin; has straight tubules and is laid down before the completion of the apical foramen.
2. Regular secondary dentin; is characterized by a slower rate of deposition and an abrupt change in the direction of the dentinal tubules.
3. Tertiary or irregular secondary (also called irritation, reparative, or reactive); dentin is laid down in response to an irritation or damage to the overlying dentin and/or enamel and this dentin has irregularly arranged and few dentinal

tubules with aging or severe damage, tertiary dentin can obliterate the pulp cavity.

STRUCTURES OF DENTIN

1. Dentinal Tubules; These tubules are perpendicular to the dentino-enamel and dentinocementum junctions the course of the dentinal tubules is curved and resembles an "S" shape. Dentinal tubules have lateral branches throughout the dentine which are termed "canaliculi".

2. Peritubular dentin; This is a transparent zone that forms the wall of the dentinal tubule.

3. Intertubular dentin; This is the region external to the peritubular dentin and it is majorly the main body of the dentin.

4. Mantle dentin; this is the external, 1st-

formed portion of the dentin beneath both the enamel and cementum.

5. Circumpulpal dentin; is the main portion of dentin i.e. it is formed after mantle dentin.

Scanned micrograph of Dentine; A, Intertubular dentin; B, Peritubular dentin; C, Dentinal tubule

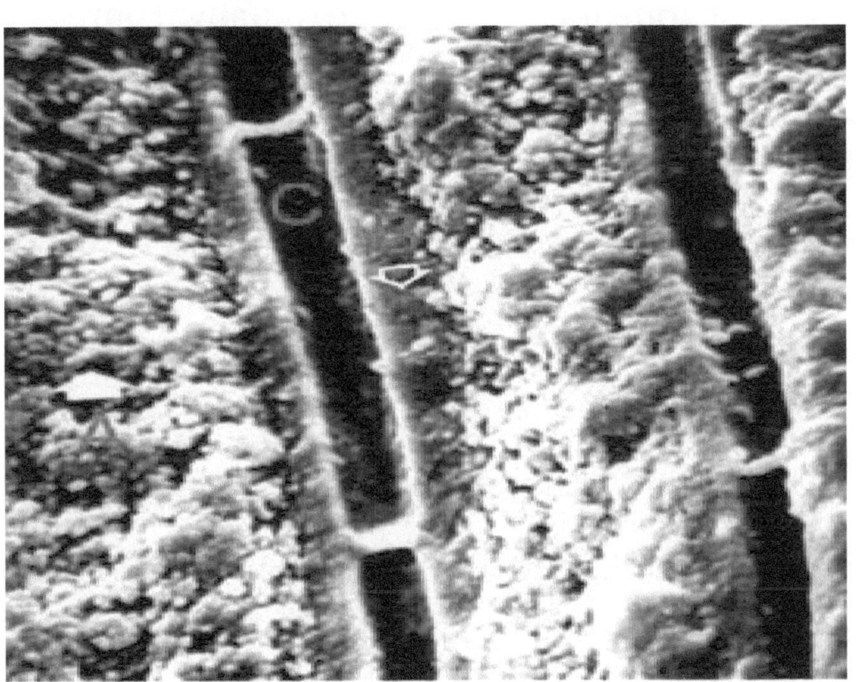

DENTINOGENESIS

The process of formation and laying down of dentin, takes place in a two-phase sequence which are: Predentin formation (Elaboration of an uncalcified organic matrix predentin) and mineralization (Crystal deposition in the form of very fine plates of hydroxyapatite, crystal deposition appears to take place radially from common centers in a so-called spherulite form).

CEMENTUM

Cementum is the bonelike tissue that covers the roots of the teeth in a thin layer. It is light yellow, in color slightly lighter than dentin.

The cementum is composed of approximately

55% organic material and 45% inorganic material; the inorganic components are mainly calcium salts. The cementum joins the enamel at the cervix of the tooth forming the cemento-enamel joint (CEJ).

In most teeth, the c e m e n t u m overlaps the enamel for a short distance. In some, the enamel meets the cementum in a sharp line. In a few, a gap may be present between the enamel and the c e m e n t u m, exposing a narrow area of root dentin. Such areas may be very sensitive to thermal, chemical, or mechanical stimuli.

The main function of cementum is to anchor the teeth to the bony walls of the tooth sockets in the periodontum. This is accomplished by the fibers of the periodontal ligament or membrane. Cementum is formed continuously throughout the life of the tooth to compensate for the loss of tooth substance because of occlusal wear and to allow for the attachment of new fibers of the periodontal ligament to the surface of the root.

THE PULP

The dental pulp, is the soft tissue inside the tooth developed from the connective tissue of the dental papilla. Within the crown, the chamber containing the dental pulp is called the pulp chamber. The coronal pulp and pulp horns are within the crown and the radicular pulp is within the root. The apical foramen is at the end or apex of the radicular pulp. Blood vessels, nerves, lymphatics cells, odontoblasts, fibroblasts, defense cells, and connective tissue pass through this area to reach the interior of the tooth.

The main function of the pulp is the formation of dentin. It furnishes nourishment to the dentin; provides sensation to the tooth; and responds to irritation, either by forming reparative secondary dentin or by becoming inflamed.

CHAPTER THREE

DEVELOPMENT OF THE JAWS

The most typical feature in the development of the head and neck is formed by the brachial or pharyngeal arches. Appear in the 4th-5th week of development, contribute to the external appearance of the embryo, and consists of bars of mesenchymal tissue separated by deep clefts called pharyngeal clefts.

Mesenchymal prominences are formed at about 42days of development mandibular prominences, maxillary prominences, and frontonasal prominence.

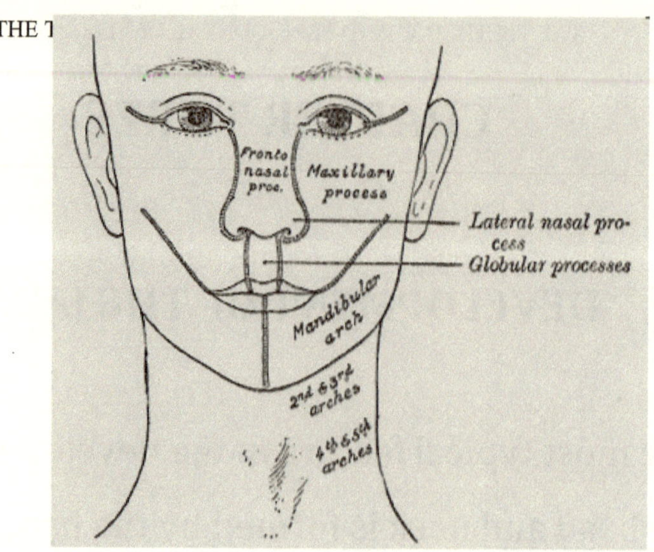

Fronto nasal proc.
Maxillary process
Lateral nasal process
Globular processes
Mandibular arch
2nd & 3rd arches
4th & 5th arches

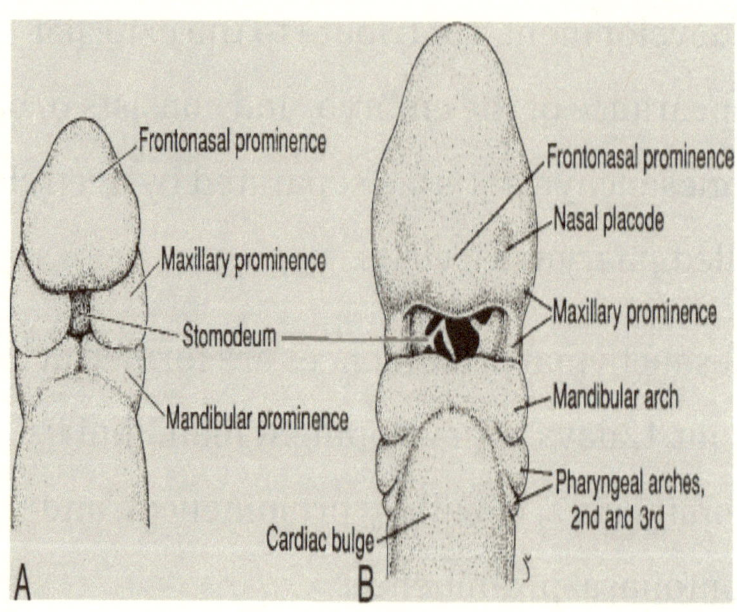

Frontonasal prominence
Maxillary prominence
Stomodeum
Mandibular prominence
A
Frontonasal prominence
Nasal placode
Maxillary prominence
Mandibular arch
Pharyngeal arches, 2nd and 3rd
Cardiac bulge
B

MANDIBLE DEVELOPMENT

Primary cartilage and Meckel's cartilage are formed around the 6th week of intra-uterine life (IUL). The dorsal end gives rise to the malleus of the middle ear, The remaining part associated with the development of the mandible includes the mandibular nerve(1st pharyngeal arch), Lingual nerve (medially), Inferior alveolar nerve (laterally) – mental & incisive nerves.

In the body of the mandible, the band of dense fibro cellular tissue lies on the lateral side of the inferior alveolar & incisive nerves. Ossification occurs at the 7th week of inta-uterine life (IUL) around the angle formed by both inferior Alveolar & incisive nerves. The alveolar bone at the bell stage of tooth development, the bone of the mandible comes in contact by the upward growth of the lateral & medial plates of the bone. Developing teeth lie in a trough of bone which later develops into small basins (alveoli).

The ramus of the mandible is produced by the spread of the ossification from the body and bone growth occurs rapidly leading to the formation of coronoid & condylar processes.

Secondary/accessory cartilages modify, further growth, occurs at various sites and they differ from the primary cartilage both in behavior & histological appearance of Condylar cartilage – largest, Coronoid cartilage and Symphyseal cartilages (two).

Symphyseal cartilages are separated from each other by connective tissue of the symphysis which enables the mandible to grow in width and disappear after birth.

Mandible at birth differs from the adult mandible, wide mandibular angle, small ramus compared with the body of poorly developed chin, and more growth after birth.

CHAPTER FOUR

TEMPO-MANDIBULAR JAW DEVELOPMENT (TMJ)

Mandibular condensation maps out the shape of the condyle, a close approximation of the condyle to the temporal region is brought about by the development of the secondary cartilage in the condylar process obliteration of the previously wide interarticular interval and articular eminence attains its typical form after the formation of the deciduous dentition.

TEMPO MANDIBULAR JAW

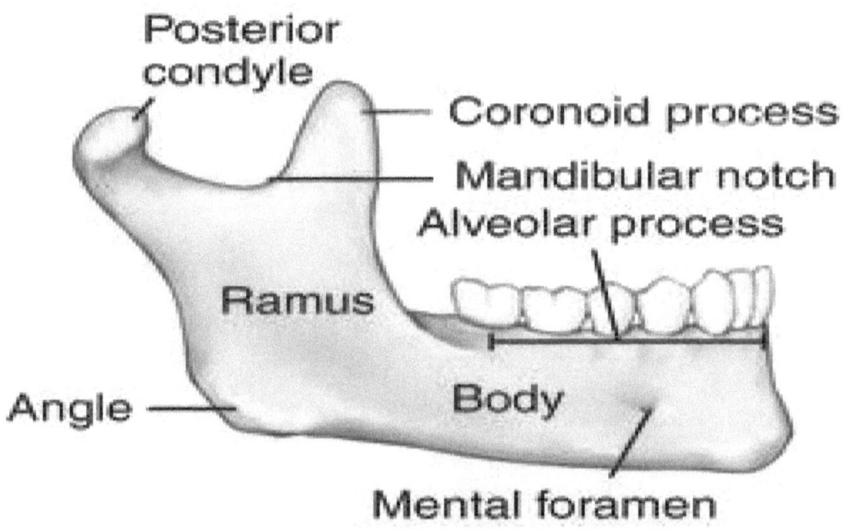

CHAPTER FIVE

MAXILLARY DEVELOPMENT

Maxillary develops from the maxillary process of the mandibular arch intramembranous like the mandible the development is affected by secondary cartilage. The ossification center appears below the infraorbital nerve giving off its anterior superior alveolar nerve.

Developing bones are arranged vertically with a convex side directed medially, developing facial & frontal processes of the premaxillary and maxillary unite with one another. Maxillary grows upward, downward, and backward with the palatal process. Secondary cartilages, zygomatic cartilage, margins of alveolar plates, mid-line of developing hard palate, and primary skeleton of the upper face – nasal cartilage.

Premaxillary is formed at the junction of the maxillary and frontonasal processes. Maxillary bone and premaxilla produce a single mass of bone – maxillary corpus (each side), incisive foramen forward to the alveolar process between the canine & lateral Incisor of both sides.

Maxillary sinus appears about the 4th month of fetal life as a small out-pocketing of the mucosa from the lateral wall of the nasal cavity separated from the developing maxillary by the cartilage of the nasal capsule, final height of the maxilla is reached when the permanent teeth have completely erupted. Sinus may be in size by extension into the alveolar process.

CHAPTER SIX
PERIODONTAL TISSUES

The periodontal tissues are fibrous connective tissue that is cellular and vascular that surrounds and support the teeth and they are collectively called the periodontium. Their main functions are to support, protect, and provide nourishment to the teeth. The periodontium consists of the cementum, alveolar process of the maxillae and mandible, periodontal ligament, and gingiva.

Periodontium Comprises Of Four Connective Tissues;

1. Two mineralized (Cementum and Alveolar bone)

2. Two fibrous (Periodontal ligament and

Lamina propria of the gingival).

PERIODONTAL LIGAMENT

The periodontal ligament is a thin, fibrous ligament that connects the tooth to the bony socket. Normally, teeth do not contact the bone directly; a tooth is suspended in its socket by the fibers of the ligament. This arrangement allows each tooth limited individual movement. The fibers act as shock absorbers to cushion the force of mastication.

DEVELOPMENT OF PERIODONTAL LIGAMENT (PDL)

The collagen fibers of the periodontal ligament develop from the cells of the dental follicle, the formation of the periodontal ligament occurs after the cells of Hertwig's epithelial root sheath have separated, forming the epithelial rests of Malassez. This separation permits the cells of the dental follicle to migrate to the external surface of the newly formed root dentin.

FUNCTIONS OF PERIODONTAL LIGAMENT

1. SUPPORTIVE:

The movement of a tooth in its socket as a result of forces acting on it during mastication or through the application of an orthodontic force leads to the compression of the periodontal ligament.

Collagen fibres in the ligament act as a cushion while the pressure of blood in the numerous blood vessels provides a hydraulic mechanism for the support of the tooth.

2. SENSORY:

The periodontal ligament through its nerve supply provides an efficient proprioceptive mechanism allowing the detection of the most delicate forces to the teeth and also a very slight displacement of the teeth.

3. NUTRITION:

The ligament transmits blood vessels which provide nutrients in other substances required by the cells of the ligament

The blood vessels also remove catabolites.

4. HOMEOSTATIC:

The cells of the periodontal ligament have the capacity to resorb and synthesize the extracellular substance of connective tissue of the ligament, alveolar bone, and cementum, thereby controlling the homeostasis of the tissues.

CELLS OF THE PERIODONTAL LIGAMENT

1. The cellular constituents of the periodontal ligament include;

- osteoblasts

- osteoclasts

- fibroblasts

- epithelial rests of Malassez

- undifferentiated mesenchymal cells

- cementoblasts

- cementoclasts

- neurovascular elements .

2. Extracellular constituents of the periodontal ligament consist of;

- collagen fibers

- oxytalan fibers

- ground substance

- nerves and vessels.

3. Synthetic cells;

- Osteoblasts

- Fibroblasts

- Cementoblasts.

4. Resorptive cells;

- Osteoclasts

- Cementoclasts.

5. Progenitor cells.

6. Epithelial rests of Malassez.

CHAPTER SEVEN

CLINICAL CORRELATIONS OF THE JAW, DENTINE AND PERIODONTAL LIGAMENT.

CLINICAL CORRELATION OF THE JAWS
1. Facial clefts
   a. Cleft lip & palate
2. No teeth, no alveolar processes
3. Unilateral growth failure → asymmetrical growth
4. Bilateral growth failure → under development of the facial structures.

CLINICAL CORRELATION OF THE DENTINE
1. Dentin hypersensitivity
2. Tooth decay involving the dentin
3. Failed tooth fillings
4. Dentin dysplasia
5. Dentin hypoplasia

CLINICAL CORRELATION OF THE PERIODONTAL LIGAMENT

1. Trauma from occlusion
2. Periodontal infections
   a. From gingiva
   b. From tooth
3. Dental prosthesis
   a. Orthodontic appliances

ABOUT THE AUTHOR

Dr. Lynda Charles, a dental surgeon, and a well-renowned researcher have done scientist and clinical research about the development of jaws, teeth, and the formation of periodontal tissue in the human oral cavity.

 Dr. Lynda has a lot of well-researched books on medical, dental, and health and this book help both the medical and dental student, nursing student, general health students, and parents.

Dr. Lynda ensures that every of his book is comprehensive and concise.